YOGA for the
New Millennium
Dhrana Reflections Off the Mat, Poems and Images

Deborah Williams

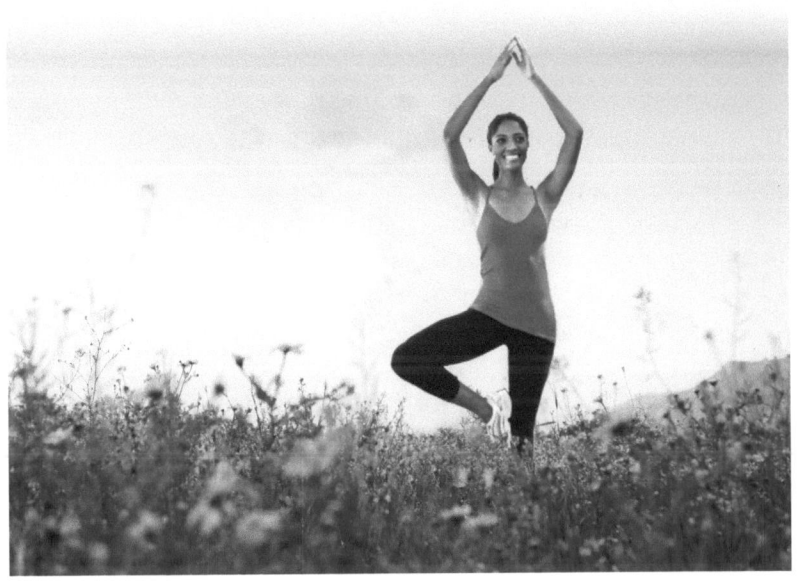

Introduction

I have learned a lot about what makes me tick. I have enjoyed the process of growing with grace into the middle years of my life. Throughout the pages of this book are various snapshots of my yoga journey expressed in poems. Enjoy.

Namaste,
D

Dedication.

To my daughter Mari, I salute and celebrate you. I think about you and your family often and you are all in my prayers. I wish for you all of the best that this world has to give. Any bumps in the road of life that you experience will pass and on the other side of what may seem like a mighty mountain you will stride downhill with grace, your head held strong and you'll be wiser for the climb up the next mountain just ahead. I hope you will never lose your caring heart and that you always find the time to tell your children how much you care about them. Also, remember to keep in touch with others who love you. I look forward to our growing old together.

With all my love,
Mom

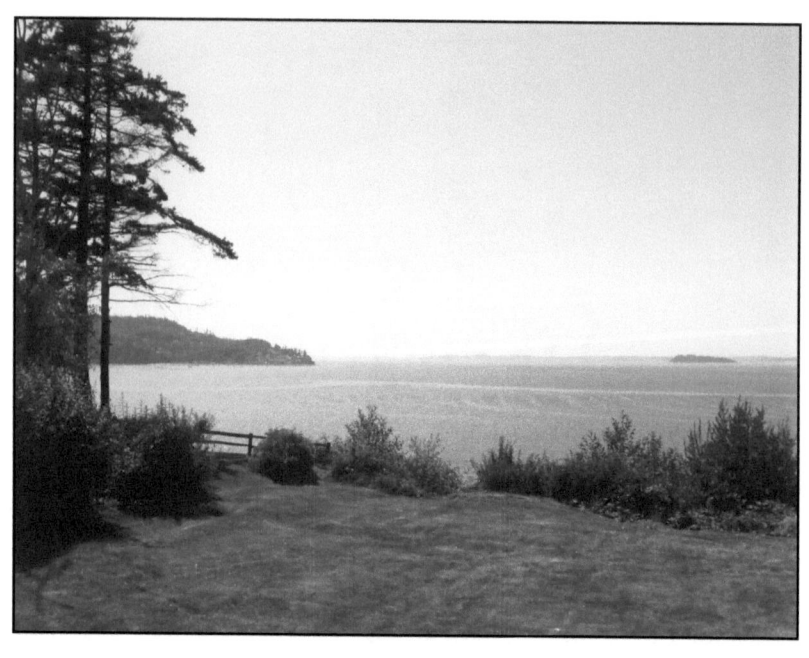

What is yoga?

Yoga is a discipline for promoting greater fullness of life.

Yesterday, I died

There in the middle of a busy intersection, not too far from home, I died.

I saw the bus and the bus saw me, but the car on the other side of the bus was not there to me.

The driver on the bus signaled me to stop, but that might have caused me to drop, so I thought I should proceed, but I died.

Within an instant the driver of the car with hair trigger instincts, saw my frame and laid on the brakes to keep me from harm.

Upon boarding the bus everyone said, "Girl you were almost dead."

It took me a minute to catch my breath and to realize what they meant

It was with a gush of emotion that I disabled my pride and realized that one second more and I would have died.

I am now convinced that without a doubt, I survived, in order to do the work that my ancestors started.

ᕈᗢ

05/12/2011 06:12 PM

I began charting a new course for the chapters of my mid-life, first, through setting my intention and writing down what I wanted to see in my future. Then building courage and taking actions towards my goals. I realize that every day is an opportunity to live anew and perhaps change just a little (or a lot). I was willing to change, grow, and learn new things about the world and about myself.

Poem #1 for WSY

He is soft to the touch but strong and deep,
no wind in his sails he drifts in his sleep.
I wonder what he holds inside with so much to share and much
more to hide.
The one who lives like an island is always alone.
Never spinning out of control or losing any of the shine on his
soul.
However, the reflection has a crack right down the center.
So, I watch and wait and tinker and toy,
I press and push and circle about,
With hope that his real self will come outside to play.

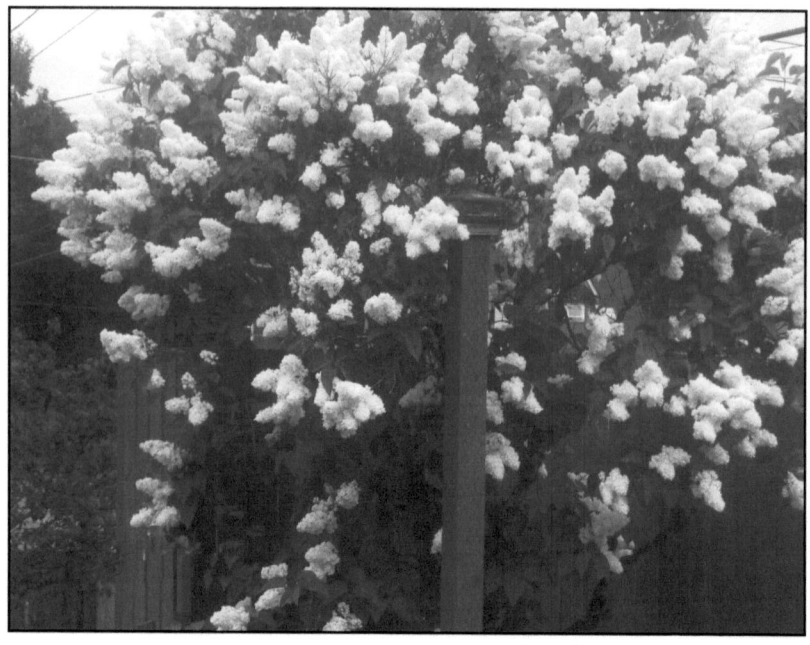

Take time to walk in the park. And listen to life. And notice that everything has its own rhythm but all coexist in harmony. Create the music of your life for all to hear and enjoy.

Love flower blooming

Love makes my heart fill with joy.
I breathe it into my soul and there it rests.
When you come close, it will find you and spring full,
like a flower blooming in the light of the sun.
Never doubt your power to nurture love inside yourself
until one comes who will shower you with the gentle rain waters
that cause your love sea to rise up from within to unite as one.
Never doubt that this was meant to be and that this love is for
you and me.

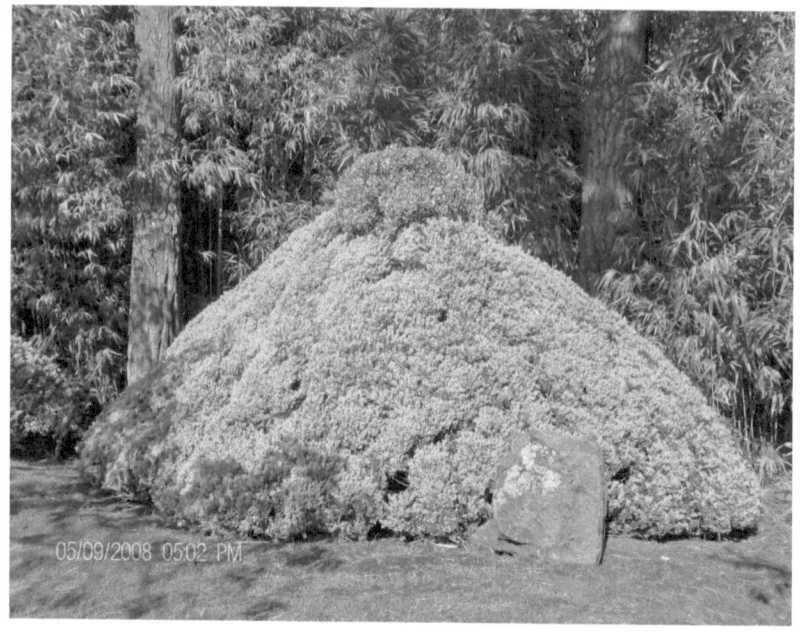

The road less travelled is the road to the inner self.

Becoming Whole Again

When I become whole, I can feel it.
The life force inside me surges towards the surface.
My soul opens and a light shines forth like no other.
I am at one with my self and my surroundings.
Today I became whole.

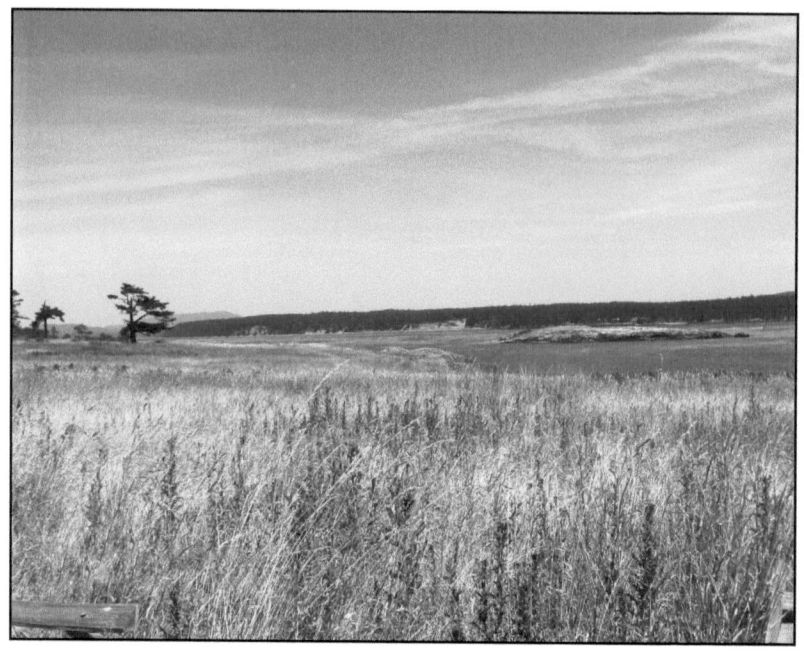

My dreams involve making myself the best person I can be and living my best life and sharing that life with others who have similar dreams (that are manifest and those that are yet to unfold).

Keep the Faith

When your life hits an all time low,
nowhere to run no place to go.
You are dealing, wheeling and borrowing the time,
closing your eyes and taking the ride.
It isn't easy oh no, oh no.
You got to pay for yesterday, today and tomorrow.
It's too late to get off or turn back or stop.
And you feel like you want to drop.
Stay cool and from deep within keep the faith.

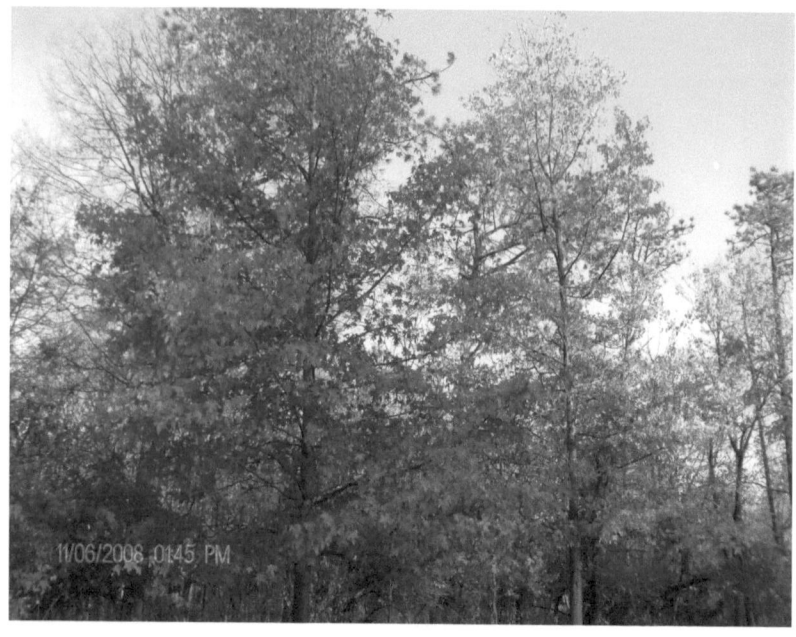

Through yoga I can take myself to a place I have never been mentally, physical and emotionally. I literally wanted to change myself from the inside out. Yoga helped me in this process.

Four – untitled

1.

I hate feeling this way, it's like everything comes inside. The shell is gone, I feel, I feel Damn it feels good.

2.

She's in the hospital today. They put a man in the same room with her. And she had to have help to use the bathroom. She came to my house when she got sick. There were no tears in our eyes. She knew I wouldn't let her down. I didn't feel special, I felt proud.

3.

I love for all of you who did not make the trip. Falling prey, they can't swallow you whole. So a bit at a time was taken. Couldn't drown your spirit. Cause you buried it in us. The pain was suffered and the wounds were deep. But this love wouldn't die.

4.

I saw a baby who died today, I felt shocked, oh! No! She couldn't have been more than three. Her home was bombed by the enemy.

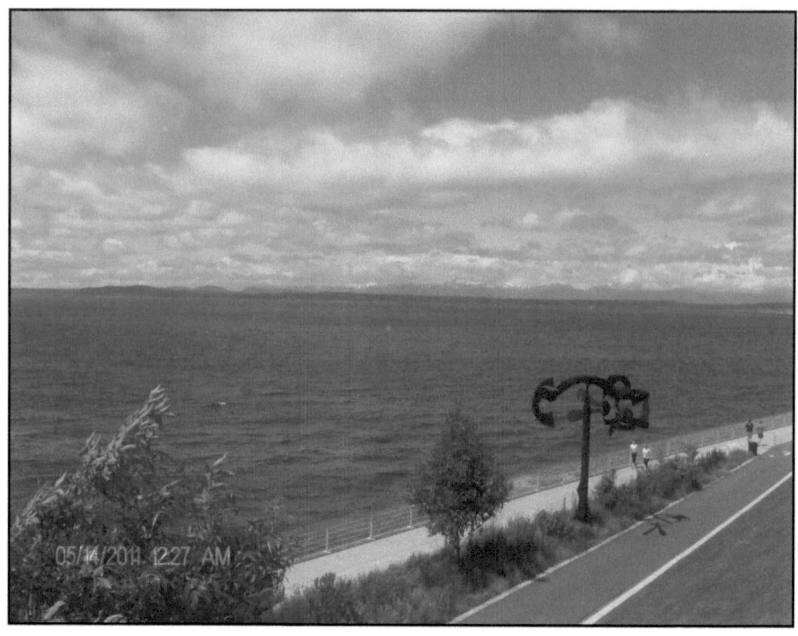

I think of yoga as a path to liberation of the mind, through overcoming limitations and fears. I learned through yoga to see fear for what it is, a mental construct that can be dismantled with time and commitment.

Miami Musing

Ticking away by the second hand,
clocking the moments.
Until we trigger the evolution of our transition,
to a new era, of self discovery and compassion.
We are all moving towards our evolved enlightenment in this
life.
[Dedicated to Valerie Y.]

05/12/2011 06:12 PM

With a forward bend, as in head to knee postures, it seems impossible at first. But over time, my body wanted to lean further into the posture and eventually it did. Inside a forward fold with my head on my knee, I focus on one thing; breathe naturally.

Feelings for Tomorrow

Make this pain go away,
make this hurt dissipate.
It is at once on and off again.
I want to smile and feel the joy,
but instead I want to take a leap of faith
into the new world of love and peace inside my mind.
There is a realm of happiness for me
detached and untouchable.

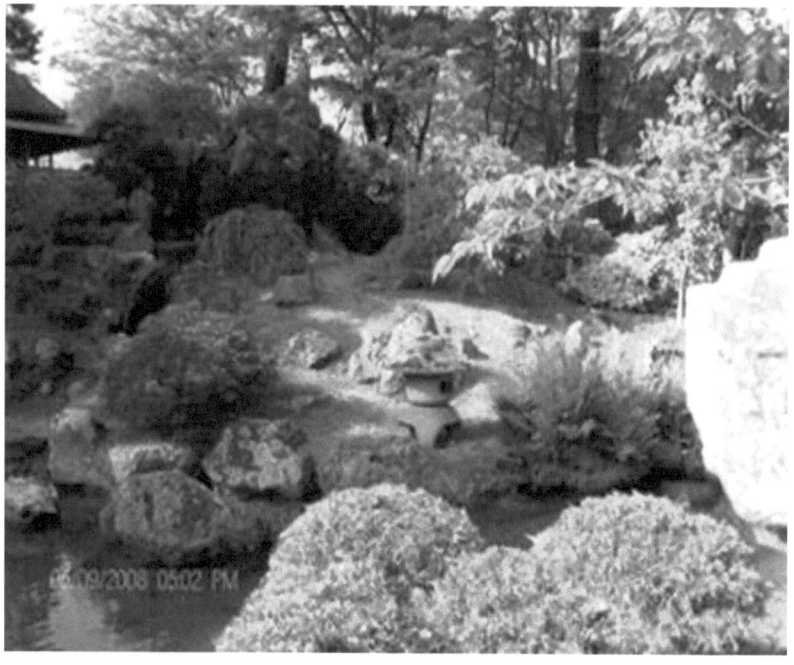

Using focused attention and changing my inner dialog, I change the feelings of doubt. I awaken and look into the mirror to see someone I love very much. I remind myself that I do not need the approval of others, but that I if I am in touch with myself, people will accept me as I am.

Opening

Writing with passion fills my soul with joy and peace.
It feels like I am the observer telling the story of my thoughts.
Taking each emotion one by one and unraveling it.
Much as a rose would unravel,
its petals to become fully open to the sun.
I unveil my inner thoughts to the light with peace
and love as my only motivation.

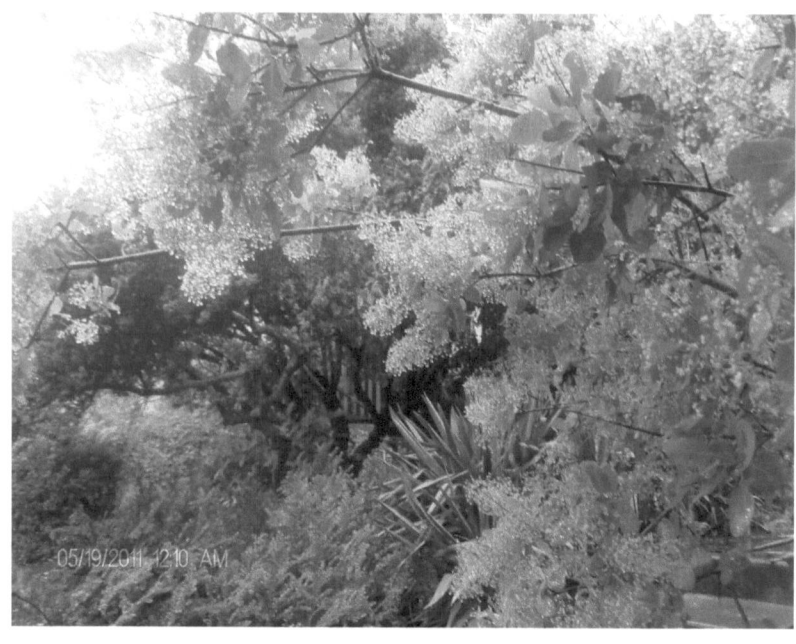

It is my wish that you find a place for yoga in your existing wellness program or that you learn to use yoga as the anchor to kick-start your program if you are starting a new one.

Grow with Grace

What does it take to grow with grace towards your ultimate
destiny?
What are the most sincere desires of ones heart?
Learning and loving each day, you discover who you really are.
How do you live with courage and determination?
Always keep an eye towards your dreams.
I think this is by staying in touch with your own reality.
In addition, realizing that in an instant this too shall pass.
Everyday I am learning as my destiny unfolds moment by moment.
I will keep you posted.

07/03/2009 01:26 PM

Faith is the seed I am sowing, wisdom is my plow. Eliminating evil karma from my deeds, words and thoughts is my weeding. Assiduity is my cow, who carries heavy burdens securely. She goes on and never retreats. She goes on but never feels sad. I am tilling like this, I am seeding like this. Eternal life is the harvest and I free myself from all suffering. – a Buddhist prayer

Boat Ride to Tortuga

The waters churn with the motion of life,
On the end of a journey aboard the Manta Ray,
With a mix of all flavors and hues,
The clamor of noise cannot break the once still joy,
Of the rocks and trees that watch patiently,
Forever in their own solemn mood,
Forever knowing there is nothing to fear,
And living in silence and grace,
Never in awe of the ever changing voices that break the
silence,
Each day but for an instant, then turn away,
They go back to the hustle of their lives,
Never really touched by the grace and freedom,
That ever waits in patience and silence,
On the boat ride to Tortuga Bay.

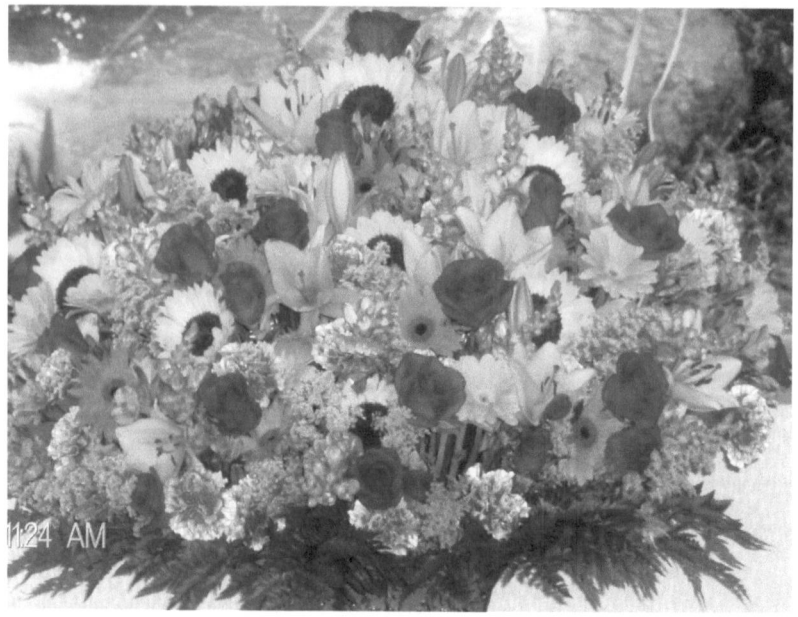

Thinking about my Nanny

9/1/09

The tears streamed down my face. Thinking it would be a disgrace to feel such sadness, regret and loss for my nanny. It is her birthday and I miss her so much. If she were here we would throw a party, with cake, ice cream and balloons. So, I turned up the music and danced for her in hope that she had time to celebrate her life even though she could not get my present.

Mary Inez

Her passing into the next realm of existence ended her suffering
in her physical body in this life. I was happy for her.

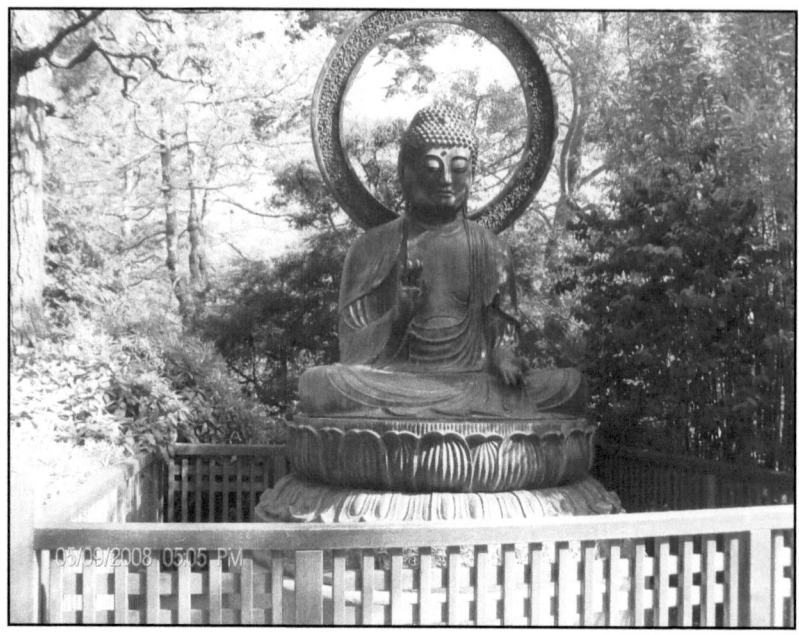

"The art of yoga begins with a code of behavior in order to build up moral conduct, mental conduct and spiritual conduct" – B. K. S. Iyengar (Light on Yoga)

Reflections on the Yoga Sutras

The yoga philosophy espoused by Patanjali,
is the challenge of living the yogic life.
It is a shift from so much focus on what is going on outside of me,
toward what I am discovering about what goes on inside of me.
It is a perfect compliment for building the discipline of the mind
and body.
This is necessary to reach deeper inward towards the creator
that abides within me.

༄

Acknowledgements

I would like to express my appreciation to the sages who have handed down the art of yoga, the teachers who shared the knowledge with me, and the students who earnestly practice to the best of their ability.

www.ingramcontent.com/pod-product-compliance
Lightning Source LLC
Chambersburg PA
CBHW050911290526
45792CB00002B/768